DAS GE

COOKBOOK

Schnitzel, Bratwurst, Strudel and other German Classics

by Franz Schulmeister

Contents

Soups, Starters & Sides

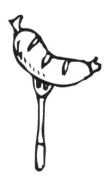

Goulash Soup
Gulaschsuppe
Preparation time: **30 min**
Cooking time: **1 h 30 min**

Ingredients:
6 Servings
- 1 ½ lbs. boneless beef chuck roast, cut in ½" cubes
- ⅓ cup lard, about 3 oz (or a blend of ½ unsalted butter and ½ canola oil)
- 1 large onion, diced
- 3 cloves garlic, crushed
- 1 tsp tomato paste
- 1 tbsp hot paprika
- 2 tbsp mild (sweet) paprika
- 1 tsp caraway seeds
- ½ cup red wine
- 4 cups beef stock
- 1 can (14.5 oz) chopped tomatoes
- 1 tsp dried marjoram
- 3 bay leaves
- 1 small bunch parsley, chopped
- ½ tsp black pepper
- 1 large carrot, peeled and diced
- 2 bell peppers, 1 green and 1 red
- 1 stick of celery, diced
- 3 medium potatoes, peeled and diced
- salt and black pepper, to taste
- sour cream to serve

1. In a large pot, on high heat, fry the beef until browned all over. Do this in batches so as not to overcrowd the pot, which will stew the meat instead of browning. Remove the beef from the pot and reduce the heat to medium low.
2. Add the onions and garlic and sauté for 5 minutes, or until softened. Stir in the tomato paste and cook for a minute. Add the paprika and caraway seeds and cook for a further minute.
3. Deglaze the pot with red wine.
4. Add the beef stock, can of tomatoes, marjoram, bay leaves, ½ the parsley, black pepper, carrot, bell peppers and celery.
5. Cover the pot with a lid and simmer for 1 hour. Stir occasionally.
6. Add the potatoes and cook for a further 25 minutes, or until the potatoes are tender.
7. Taste and adjust the seasoning with salt and pepper if desired.
8. Serve with a dollop of sour cream and a sprinkling of parsley.

Chicken Broth with Pancake Strips
Flädlesuppe

Preparation time: **30 min**
Cooking time: **1 h 30 min**

Ingredients:
4 Servings
For the broth
- 2.2 lbs. skinless, bone-in chicken thighs
- 4 carrots, halved
- 1 stick celery, halved
- ½ small (about 8 oz) celeriac, peeled and quartered
- 1 large onion, quartered
- 2 large cloves garlic, halved
- 1 tsp dried thyme
- 10 black peppercorns
- 1 tsp kosher salt
- 1 clove
- 4 bay leaves
- 1 bunch parsley, stalks only (leaves reserved for finishing soup)
- 6 ¼ cups water
- 2 tbsp chives, chopped
- 2 tbsp parsley, chopped

For the pancakes
- 1 ½ cups all-purpose flour
- 3 eggs
- 2 cups whole milk
- ½ tsp salt, or to taste
- pinch of nutmeg
- oil for greasing the pan

1. Add all the ingredients for the broth, except the chicken and fresh herbs, to a large pot and bring to the boil.
2. Add the chicken, reduce to a simmer and cover with a lid. Cook for 15 to 20 minutes, or until the chicken is cooked through and almost falling off the bone.
3. Remove the chicken and shred all the meat off the bones. Skim off any scum that may have risen to the surface.
4. Add the bones back to the broth and simmer, with the lid on, for another hour. The longer the broth is simmered, the more the flavor will develop. If you have the time, gently simmer for up to 3 hours. Skim the surface of any scum from time to time.
5. Beat the egg with the milk, salt and nutmeg. Gradually add to the flour, whisking with an electric beater until smooth. Leave to rest for about ½ hour.

6. Strain the broth through a fine sieve or muslin cloth and pour back into the cleaned pot. Taste and season with extra salt and pepper if desired. Discard the bones and vegetables.
7. Add the shredded chicken and half the fresh herbs to the broth and place the pot on low heat to keep the broth warm whilst you prepare the pancakes.
8. Heat a crepe pan or frying pan on medium heat and brush with a little oil. Pour enough batter to coat the pan and make a thin crepe. Tilt the pan to spread the batter evenly. Cook until set and then flip and cook the other side. Remove from the pan and immediately roll up into a cylinder. Repeat until all the batter is used.
9. Slice the pancakes crosswise into ¼ inch strips. Keep them rolled up.
10. Distribute the pancake rolls between the soup bowls. A broad, shallow soup bowl is best.
11. Pour over the broth and shredded chicken, and sprinkle with the remaining fresh herbs.

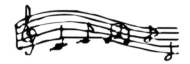

Berliner Potato Soup
Berliner Kartoffelsuppe

Preparation time: **15 min**
Cooking time: **40 min**

Ingredients:
6 Servings

- 4 tbsp canola oil
- 5 oz slab smoked bacon, diced
- 3 onions, diced
- 2 cloves garlic, minced
- 2 large carrots, peeled and diced
- 1 leek, diced
- ½ celeriac (celery root, peeled and diced
- 4 cups (2 pts.) vegetable stock
- 2 ½ lbs. Yukon Gold potatoes, peeled and diced
- ½ tsp caraway seeds, ground
- 1 tbsp fresh marjoram, or 1 tsp dried
- 4 bay leaves, preferably fresh
- 10 black peppercorns
- 1 small bunch parsley, chopped
- ¼ tsp nutmeg
- 5 frankfurters, sliced into thin rings
- 1 onion, sliced
- kosher salt and freshly ground black pepper, to taste
- ½ cup cream (optional)

1. Heat 3 tbsp oil in a large pot. Add the bacon and onions and sauté until onions are softened. Add garlic and sauté for another minute.
2. Add the carrots, leek and celeriac and cook for another 3 minutes.
3. Pour in the stock, add the potatoes, caraway, marjoram, bay leaves, peppercorns and ½ the parsley.
4. Bring to the boil and then immediately reduce to a simmer. Place the lid on the pot and simmer the soup for 30 minutes, or until the potatoes are tender.
5. Using a slotted spoon remove ⅓ of the vegetables to a bowl.
6. Use a hand stick blender to blend the soup, in the pot, until smooth.
7. Return the vegetables back to the soup and add nutmeg. Taste and add salt and pepper if desired. Re-heat the soup and keep warm.
8. Sauté the frankfurter rings and sliced onion in a tablespoon of oil until the onions and frankfurter rings are nicely browned and cooked through.
9. Optional: add cream and simmer the soup for 2 minutes to re-heat.
10. Spoon the sautéed onions and frankfurter on the soup and sprinkle with parsley.

Red Cabbage with Apple
Apfel-Rotkohl

Preparation time: **15 min**
Cooking time: **55 min**

Ingredients:
6 Servings

- 2 tbsp lard or butter
- 1 onion, halved and sliced
- 1 large red cabbage, quartered, cored and thinly sliced
- 1 Granny Smith apple, peeled and grated
- ½ cup golden raisins, optional
- ¼ tsp ground nutmeg
- ¼ tsp ground allspice
- ½ tsp ground cloves
- 1 tsp ground cinnamon
- 1 tbsp brown sugar, or to taste
- ½ cup red wine
- ¼ cup red wine vinegar
- 2 cups clear apple juice or water
- 2 bay leaves
- salt and black pepper, to taste1

1. Heat the lard in a large Dutch oven or heavy-bottomed pot on medium heat.
2. Sauté the onions until softened, about 5 minutes.
3. Add the cabbage, apple and (optional) raisins, stir to combine and sauté for 5 minutes.
4. Stir in the spices, bay leaves and sugar, and sauté for 3 minutes. Season with salt and pepper, to taste.
5. Pour in the red wine, vinegar, apple juice and bay leaves, and bring to the boil.
6. Reduce the heat to low and simmer with the lid on for 40 minutes, or until the cabbage is tender.
7. Check the pot about 15 minutes before completing the cooking and if the cabbage is too moist, continue cooking with the lid off.
8. Taste and adjust the seasoning with salt and pepper, if desired.
9. Serve hot immediately or chill for re-heating later.

Potato Salad

Kartoffelsalat

Preparation time: **15 min**
Cooking time: **20 min**

Ingredients:
4-6 Servings

- 1 ½ lbs. Yukon gold or red skinned potatoes, cut into approx. ¾" cubes
- 1 cup beef or chicken stock, hot
- 5 oz smoked slab bacon, cut into ¼" cubes
- 6 tbsp canola oil
- 2 tbsp cider vinegar
- 1 tsp Dijon mustard
- ½ tsp white sugar, or to taste
- ½ tsp fine sea salt, or to taste
- ½ tsp freshly ground black pepper, or to taste
- 1 large dill pickle, cut into ¼" cubes
- 2 green onions, ¼" slices
- 1 small onion, finely diced
- 2 tbsp fresh chives, chopped
- 2 tbsp fresh flat leaf (Italian) parsley, roughly chopped
- 10 cherry tomatoes, halved
- sea salt and freshly ground black pepper, to taste

1. Cook the potatoes in salted boiling water until just tender.
2. Drain the potatoes, return them to the pot and pour over the hot beef stock. Set aside to cool and for the stock to be absorbed by the potatoes. If the potatoes are not completely covered by the stock, use a wooden spoon to carefully turn them so that they all get to absorb the stock.
3. Fry the bacon in a little oil until crispy. Drain and set aside to cool.
4. Add the canola oil, vinegar, mustard, sugar, salt and pepper to a large bowl and whisk until thoroughly combined.
5. Add the bacon, pickle, green onions, onion, chives and parsley to the dressing and stir to combine.
6. Drain off any stock that has not been absorbed by the potatoes and add them to the dressing.
7. Add the tomatoes and gently toss all the ingredients together.
8. Check the seasoning and add salt and pepper if desired.
9. Refrigerate for 1 – 2 hours before serving.

Potato Fritters with Applesauce
Kartoffelpuffer mit Apfelmus

Preparation time: **min**
Cooking time: **30 min**

Ingredients:
4 Servings
For the applesauce
- 3 cooking apples (about 1 ¾ lbs.), peeled, cored & diced
- juice of 1 lemon
- zest of 1 lemon, finely grated
- 1 cup water, or clear apple juice
- 2 tbsp sugar, or to taste
- 2 whole cloves
- ½ stick cinnamon, or ½ tsp cinnamon powder
- 1 tsp vanilla extract

For the fritters
- 4 lbs. potatoes, peeled
- 2 large onions, finely grated
- 2 large eggs, beaten
- 3 – 4 tbsp potato or all-purpose flour
- 2 tsp salt, or to taste
- Freshly ground black pepper, to taste
- ½ cup lard or canola oil, or as needed to fry fritters
- sour cream or crème fraiche (optional)

1. Add all the ingredients for the applesauce to a saucepan. Place the lid on and simmer for 15 minutes, or until the apples are tender.
2. Remove the cinnamon stick and cloves. Puree in the saucepan using a hand stick blender, until smooth. If the applesauce is still too liquid, cook with the lid off until you have the desired consistency. Set aside.
3. Coarsely grate the potatoes. Place in a dish towel and squeeze out excess liquid.
4. Finely grate, or puree, the onions. Combine in a bowl with the potato and egg and mix together. Season with salt and pepper to taste.
5. Gradually mix in flour until the mixture stiffens and holds together. Chill for ½ hour.
6. Divide the potato mixture into 16 portions and form into balls. Flatten each ball using a spatula or a damp hand.
7. Heat the lard or oil in a heavy-bottomed skillet or frying pan. Fry the fritters, in batches, until cooked through, and nicely browned and crispy on both sides. Remove to kitchen paper to drain off excess fat. Keep warm.
8. Serve with applesauce and (optional)a dollop sour cream. The applesauce can be served hot or cold, according to preference.

Cucumber Salad
Gurkensalat

Preparation time: **10 min + 1 - 2 h fridge time**
Cooking time: **0 min**

Ingredients:
4 Servings

- 2 medium English cucumbers (about 2 lbs.), peeled & very thinly sliced
- 1 small white onion, peeled & very thinly sliced
- ½ cup fresh dill, chopped
- 2 tbsp fresh chives, chopped

For a vinaigrette dressing
- 3 tbsp canola or sunflower oil
- 3 tbsp white wine vinegar
- 1 tsp sugar, or to taste
- 1 tsp sea salt, or to taste
- ½ tsp freshly ground black pepper

For a creamy dressing
- 1 tbsp white wine vinegar
- ½ - 1 tsp sugar, or to taste
- 2 tsp extra virgin olive oil
- ½ tbsp Dijon mustard
- 2 cloves garlic, mashed (optional)
- ½ cup sour cream or crème fraiche
- sea salt and freshly ground black pepper, to taste

1. The cucumbers and onion should be sliced very thinly, preferably using a mandolin. Otherwise use a sharp knife and slice as thinly as possible.
2. Add the cucumber, onion, dill and chives to a bowl and mix together.
3. For a vinaigrette dressing: add the oil, vinegar, sugar, salt and pepper to a bowl and whisk together. Pour over the cucumber mixture and toss together. Cover with plastic wrap and refrigerate for at least 2 hours before serving. The salad can be served chilled from the fridge or allowed to come to room temperature and then served.
4. For a creamy dressing: add the vinegar and sugar to a bowl and whisk to dissolve the sugar. Whisk in the olive oil, mustard and garlic until combined. Whisk in the sour cream. Taste and season with salt and pepper to taste. Pour over the cucumber mixture and combine. Cover with plastic wrap and refrigerate for an hour before serving. The salad can be served chilled from the fridge or allowed to come to room temperature and then served.

Bavarian Radish Salad
Bayerischer Radieschen-Salat

Preparation time: **20 min**

Cooking time: **0 min**

Ingredients:

4 Servings

- 1 Daikon radish (or 2 icicle radishes), peeled & thinly sliced
- 1 bunch red globe radishes, thinly sliced
- 1 red onion, peeled & thinly sliced
- 1 bunch dill, chopped (reserve some for garnish)
- 2 tbsp chives, chopped (reserve some for garnish)
- 1 tbsp fresh horseradish, grated (optional)
- 1 cup (6 oz) cherry tomatoes, halved
- 2 tbsp red wine or cider vinegar
- 1 tbsp medium-hot German mustard (use sweet mustard if using horseradish)
- 1 tsp white sugar (or honey)
- 4 tbsp canola oil (or olive oil)
- salt and freshly ground black pepper, to taste

---

1. Using a mandolin to slice the Daikon and red radishes will give the best results of thin, evenly sliced radishes. Alternatively use a very sharp knife to slice the radishes. Add to a colander with a ½ a teaspoon of salt and toss to mix. Set aside.
2. Add the vinegar, mustard and sugar to a bowl and mix together. Add the oil and whisk until well combined. Taste and season with salt and pepper.
3. Press excess liquid from the radishes, if any, and add to a large bowl.
4. Add the fresh onion, herbs and horseradish (optional) and mix together.
5. Add the tomatoes, pour over the dressing and toss to coat the ingredients well.
6. The flavors will develop and combine if the salad is left to marinate for about 15 minutes, in or out of the fridge.
7. Serve garnished with a sprinkling of dill and chives.

Bavarian Bread Dumplings
Semmelknödel

Preparation time: **30 min**
Cooking time: **20 min**

Ingredients:
4 Servings

- 1 lb. stale white bread slices, or bread rolls
- 2 cups warm milk
- 1 tbsp butter
- 1 onion, finely diced
- 1 medium bunch parsley, finely chopped
- 2 eggs, whisked
- 1 tbsp sour cream or crème fraiche
- ¼ tsp nutmeg
- salt and black pepper, to taste
- 2 tbsp all-purpose flour, or as needed
- salted water for cooking dumplings (alternatively use vegetable stock)

1. Slice the bread into pieces. Add to a bowl, pour over warm milk and cover. Soak for 30 – 40 minutes.
2. Heat the butter in a pan on medium heat. Sauté the onions until softened, about 8 minutes. Stir in the parsley. Set aside to cool.
3. Whisk together the eggs, sour cream, nutmeg, salt and pepper. Add to the soaked bread and stir to combine.
4. Stir in the cooked onion and parsley mixture. Knead until the dough is well combined.
5. If the dough is too wet and sticky, gradually add flour until you have a firm dough.
6. Form the dough into 8 balls using lightly-floured hands.
7. Bring a large pot of salted water to the boil.
8. Reduce to a simmer and add the dumplings. Cook for 15 – 20 minutes, or until done. The dumplings will float to the surface when they are done.
9. Remove the dumplings with a slotted spoon and place on kitchen paper to drain.

Sauerkraut with White Wine
Weinsauerkraut

Preparation time: **10 min**
Cooking time: **29 min**

Ingredients:
4 Servings

- 2 tbsp butter
- 3 medium onions, diced
- 1 jar (16 oz) sauerkraut, drained
- 6 juniper berries, lightly crushed
- 3 bay leaves
- ½ tsp caraway seeds
- ½ tsp freshly ground black pepper, or to taste
- 1 cup white wine
- 2 sweet apples, coarsely grated
- 1 tsp sugar, or to taste (optional)
- 2 tbsp crisp smoked bacon bits (optional)

1. Melt the butter in a saucepan on medium heat.
2. Add the onions and sauté until softened, about 8 minutes.
3. Add the sauerkraut, juniper berries, bay leaves, caraway seeds, pepper and wine. Simmer for 20 minutes.
4. Add the apple and (optional) sugar and simmer for another 10 minutes. If needed, add a little water if the sauerkraut gets too dry.
5. Optional: stir in the bacon bits and heat through for a minute.
6. Pick out the bay leaves and juniper berries, and serve.

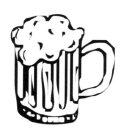

Farmhouse Sourdough Rye Bread
Bauernbrot

Preparation time: **3 h + 2 days**
Cooking time: **45 min**

Ingredients:

Servings: makes 2 large loaves

For the starter dough
- 4 cups (2 pts.) warm water (110° F - just above body temp.)
- 2 tbsp granulated white sugar
- 1 ½ oz compressed fresh yeast, or 2 tbsp active dry yeast
- 4 cups all-purpose flour

For the dough
- 4 cups all-purpose flour
- 8 cups rye flour
- 1 tsp granulated white sugar
- 1 tbsp salt
- 2 cups warm water (110° F - just above body temp.)

---

1. The first step is to prepare the starter dough. Add the warm water to a large glass or porcelain bowl and stir in the sugar. Crumble the fresh yeast into the water (or the dry yeast) and stir to dissolve. Gradually add the flour and mix until you have no lumps. NB Always check the expiry date of the yeast. It may not activate if past it's use-by date!

2. Cover with a dish cloth or oiled plastic wrap, and leave at room temperature (away from any draughts) to prove for 24 hours.

3. After 24 hours give the dough a good mix and then leave to prove, covered, for another 24 hours.

4. Sift together in a large bowl the all-purpose flour, rye flour, sugar and salt. Add to the bowl of a stand mixer with the dough hook fitted.

5. Add the dough starter and one cup of water to the stand mixer bowl and mix for a minute. Gradually add the second cup of warm water mixing on medium speed until the dough comes together, about 4 to 5 minutes. Use only as much of the second cup of water as needed. The dough should be soft, not soggy.

6. Remove the dough to a counter-top dusted with flour. Knead for 10 to 15 minutes, until you have a smooth and elastic dough. Use the heel of your hand to knead the dough, pushing the dough away from yourself. Fold back the dough and push back again with the heel of your hand. Repeat until done dusting the counter with flour, as needed. It also helps to prevent the dough sticking to your hands if you dust them with flour.

7.   Form the dough into a ball and place in a large bowl. Cover with a dish cloth or a piece of oiled plastic wrap. Leave to rise in a warm, draught-free place until doubled in size, about 2 to 3 hours.
8.   Line a baking sheet with a silicon baking mat (preferred) or kitchen parchment paper brushed with oil.
9.   Tip the dough onto a flour-dusted counter top and knead for about 5 minutes to activate the gluten. Form into two oval shapes and place on the prepared baking sheets. Leave to rise for an hour.
10.   Pre-heat the oven to 390° F. Place a baking pan at the bottom of the oven to heat up.
11.   Cut 3 or 4 deep slashes across the loaf using a sharp knife (dip the blade in hot water to stop it from sticking).
12.   Remove the baking pan from the oven, half-fill with boiling water and return to the oven. The steam will help form a lovely crust.
13.   Bake the bread for about 45 – 60 minutes, or until done. To test if the loaf is done, tap the base of the loaf with your knuckles. If it sounds hollow, it's done. If not bake for another 5 minutes.
14.   Remove from the oven and place on a wire rack to cool for 5 – 10 minutes before serving.

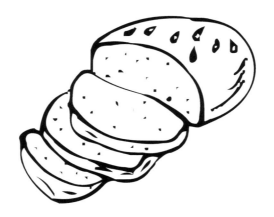

Main Courses

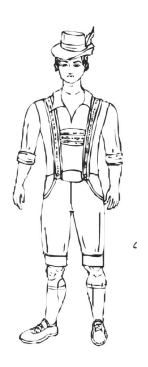

Fish Cakes with Herb Sauce
Fischfrikadellen mit Grüner Soße

Preparation time: **30 min**
Cooking time: **12 min**

Ingredients:
4 Servings

- 2 medium floury potatoes, peeled & grated
- ½ white onion, grated
- 10 oz white fish fillets, deboned & skinned
- 5 oz smoked salmon fillets, deboned & skinned
- 2 tbsp all-purpose flour for dusting, or as needed
- sea salt and freshly ground black pepper, to taste
- ½ cup olive oil for frying, or as needed

For the sauce

- 1 ½ cups (about 2 oz) fresh herbs (parsley, chives, dill or tarragon and a choice of chervil, marjoram, basil, borage, garden cress)
- ½ white onion, diced
- 3 tbsp quark (alternatively use sour cream or plain Greek-style yogurt)
- 2 tbsp mayonnaise
- 2 tsp German mustard, sweet or medium-hot
- 2 free-range eggs, hard-boiled and chopped

1. Wrap the grated potato in a dish cloth and squeeze to remove as much moisture as possible. Mix together with the grated onion. Season with salt and pepper.
2. Season the fish fillets with freshly ground black pepper and salt (remember the smoked fish will be salty). Add to a food processor bowl. Using the pulse button, blend to a coarse paste. It should be smooth but still with a little texture. Mix with the grated potato and onion.
3. Using your hands form the mixture into 8 balls. Flatten the balls with the palm of your hand to form cakes about 1 ½ inches thick. Place in the fridge, covered with plastic wrap, for about 15 minutes to firm up.
4. Clean the bowl of the food processor. Add the fresh herbs and blend until finely chopped.
5. Add the diced onion, quark, mayonnaise, mustard and chopped eggs, and pulse until you have a coarse puree. It should still have texture and not be smooth. Season with salt and black pepper to taste and remove to a serving bowl.
6. Remove fish cakes from the fridge and lightly dust both sides with flour.

7. Heat the oil in a large skillet or frying pan on medium heat. Shallow fry the fish cakes (in about ½-inch of oil), in batches, for about 3 minutes on each side, or until cooked through, crispy and golden brown. Remove to kitchen paper to drain excess oil. Allow the oil to re-heat before frying the next batch of fish cakes.
8. Serve warm with the herb sauce.

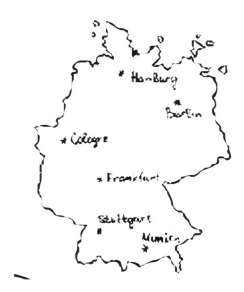

Salmon on Wine Sauerkraut
Lachs auf Wein-Sauerkraut

Preparation time: **30 min**

Cooking time: **30 min**

Ingredients:

4 Servings

- 8 skinless salmon fillets (about 3 ½ oz each)
- sea salt and freshly ground black pepper, to taste
- 1 un-waxed lemon, juiced
- 1 stick (4 oz.) salted butter, melted (reserve some for greasing the baking dish)
- 14 oz wine sauerkraut
- zest of 1 lemon, sliced into thin strips
- 2 tbsp fresh chervil, chopped
- 1 ⅓ cups crème fraiche
- 3 tbsp whipping cream
- 1 cup dry white wine, such as Riesling

1. Pre-heat the oven to 350° F (fan).
2. Grease a porcelain baking dish with butter.
3. Brush the salmon fillets with lemon juice and season with salt and pepper.
4. Tip the sauerkraut into a bowl and loosen with a fork. Drain off any excess liquid.
5. Add the butter to a saucepan on medium heat to brown (beurre noisette). Whisk the butter as it melts and begins to foam. As the foam subsides the butter will begin to brown. Remove from the heat just as the butter becomes light brown. Be careful as the butter will burn quickly at this stage.
6. Cover the baking dish loosely with a layer of half the sauerkraut. Sprinkle over ½ the lemon zest and 1 tablespoon chervil.
7. Place a layer of four salmon fillets on the sauerkraut. Pour half the browned butter over the salmon.
8. Repeat with another layer of sauerkraut, lemon zest, chervil, salmon and butter.
9. Mix together the crème fraiche, cream and wine. Season with salt and pepper to taste. Pour over the salmon.
10. Bake in the pre-heated oven for 30 minutes.
11. Serve immediately from the oven.

Berliner Curry Sausage
Berliner Currywurst

Preparation time: **15 min**
Cooking time: **30 min**

Ingredients:
4 Servings

- 1 tbsp peanut or vegetable oil
- 2 large onions, sliced
- 2 tbsp mild curry powder
- ½ tsp chili powder, or to taste
- 1 tbsp smoked paprika
- ¼ tsp freshly ground black pepper
- 1 bay leaf
- ¼ tsp powdered cinnamon (optional)
- 2 (14 oz) cans chopped tomatoes
- 1 cup tomato ketchup
- 4 tbsp Worcestershire sauce
- 1 tbsp mild German mustard
- 2 tbsp brown sugar
- 3 tbsp pineapple juice or 2 tbsp apple puree/sauce (optional)
- salt, to taste
- 4 knockwurst (knackwurst) or bratwurst

1. Heat the oil in a saucepan on medium heat. Add the onions and cook for 8 minutes, or until softened.
2. Add the spices and bay leaf and cook for a further 2 minutes, stirring.
3. Add the cans of tomato, ketchup, Worcestershire sauce, mustard, sugar and (optional) pineapple juice or apple puree. Stir to combine thoroughly and cook on a gentle simmer for 10 minutes, or until thickened. Taste and add salt and pepper as needed.
4. Remove the bay leaf and puree in a countertop blender until smooth. Strain through a sieve and return to a clean saucepan.
5. Make several shallow cuts into the sausage on both sides. Fry the sausages in a pan with a little oil until cooked through and nicely browned. Turn several times during cooking.
6. Heat the sauce whilst cooking the sausages.
7. Transfer the sausages to a warm serving plate and cover with the warm sauce. Optional: sprinkle a little curry powder over the sauce.
8. Serve with a sliced mini baguette or fried onions and French fries.

Spatchcock Roast Chicken
Flaches Brathendl

Preparation time: **15 min**

Cooking time: **1 h**

Ingredients:

4 Servings

- 1 free-range chicken, about 3.5 pounds
- juice of 1 lemon
- zest of 1 lemon, finely chopped
- 2 tsp salt, or to taste
- ½ tsp freshly ground black pepper, or to taste
- 2 tsp smoked paprika
- 2 tsp dried thyme
- 2 tsp dried oregano
- ½ tsp dried rosemary
- 1 tbsp dried parsley
- 1 tbsp extra virgin olive oil
- 6 cloves garlic, crushed
- ½ stick (2 oz / 4 tbsp) butter, softened
- ¼ cup chicken stock
- ¼ cup white wine (e.g. Riesling, gewürztraminer)

---

1. To spatchcock (cut and flatten) the chicken:
   a. Place chicken breast-side down, with the legs towards you.
   b. Using a large, sharp kitchen knife or preferably kitchen shears (or sturdy scissors), cut up along each side of the parson's nose and along the backbone to remove it, cutting through the rib bones.
   c. Open the chicken out and turn over. Press down firmly with the heel of your hand on the breastbone until you hear a crack (that is the wishbone) and the chicken lies flat.
   d. Tuck the wings back under the breasts.
2. Pre-heat the oven to 350° F.
3. To a mixing bowl add the lemon juice, lemon zest and all the herbs and spices. Whisk together.
4. Whisk in the olive oil, garlic and softened butter until well combined. If the mixture is too loose (runny) place in the fridge until it firms up. This makes it easier to spread on the chicken.
5. Rub ⅓ of the mixture to the underside of the chicken. Rub the remaining butter mixture over the breast side of the chicken.
6. Pour the chicken stock and wine into the roasting pan and place the wire rack in.
7. Place the chicken breast-side up on the wire rack. Roast for 50 – 60 minutes, or until a temperature probe inserted into the thickest part

of the thigh reads 165° F (75° C). If you don't have a temperature probe, insert a skewer into the thickest part of the thigh and if the juices run clear the chicken is cooked.

8. Baste the chicken with the pan juices every 15 minutes or so.
9. If you want the skin extra crispy place the chicken about 3 inches under the oven's overhead grill (on high) until it reaches the desired crispiness. Keep your eye on the chicken as it will burn very quickly under the grill.
10. The pan juices can be used as the base for making a sauce, after skimming off excess fat.

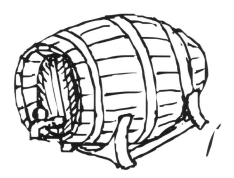

Meatballs and Sauerkraut
Buletten und Sauerkraut

Preparation time: **30 min**

Cooking time: **25 min**

Ingredients:

6 Servings

For the buletten

- 2 slices stale bread
- ½ cup milk
- ¾ lb. lean ground beef
- ¾ lb. ground pork
- 2 eggs, beaten
- 1 onion, finely chopped or minced
- 1 small bunch parsley, finely chopped (reserve some for garnish)
- 2 cloves garlic, minced
- 1 tbsp mustard
- 1 tsp dried marjoram
- 1 tsp dried thyme
- 1 tsp paprika
- 1 tsp freshly ground black pepper
- salt, to taste
- 2 tbsp lard, or ½ butter and ½ canola oil

For the sauerkraut

- 1 tsp extra virgin olive oil
- 1 tsp caraway seeds
- 3 cups (16 oz) sauerkraut, drained
- ½ cup crème fraiche
- 2 tbsp chives, chopped

1. Soak the bread in milk for about 10 minutes. Squeeze the excess milk from the bread after soaking.
2. Add all the ingredients for the meatballs to a large bowl and mix with your hands until well combined. Place the bowl, covered with plastic wrap, in the fridge for 10 minutes to firm up the mixture and make it easier to shape.
3. Remove the mixture from the fridge, divide into 12 and form into balls using damp hands (it makes it easier to handle the sticky mixture). Flatten the balls to form patties about 1 inch thick.
4. Heat the lard in a large, heavy-bottomed skillet over medium heat. Fry the meatballs for about 5 minutes on each side, or until cooked and nicely browned. Do this in batches so as not to overcrowd the pan and lower the temperature. Set aside and cover with aluminum foil to keep warm.

5. Warm the olive oil in a saucepan on medium-low heat. Add the caraway seeds for gently fry for a 1 – 2 minutes, or until the seeds start to become aromatic. Add the sauerkraut and cook until warm.
6. Remove the pan from the heat and allow to cool for a minute. Stir in the crème fraiche and chopped chives.
7. Add the sauerkraut to a warm serving plate, place the meatballs on top and sprinkle with parsley.

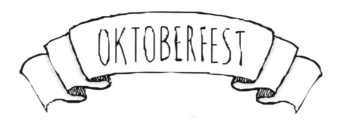

Berliner Pork Hock with Pea Puree
Berliner Eisbein mit Erbsenpüree

Preparation time: **30 min**

Cooking time: **2 h**

Ingredients:

2   Servings

For the pork hock (knuckle)

- 2 meaty cured pork hock (knuckle)
- 1 large onion, quartered
- 1 carrot, roughly chopped
- 1 stick celery, roughly chopped
- 1 small bunch parsley (including stalks)
- 3 bay leaves
- 10 peppercorns
- 5 allspice berries

For the pea puree

- ½ stick (4 tbsp) butter
- 1.5 oz (about 3 ½ tbsp) diced bacon or smoked ham
- 1 shallot, finely diced
- ½ carrot, finely diced
- ½ stick celery, finely diced
- ¼ tsp marjoram
- ¼ tsp thyme
- ½ cup Noilly Prat vermouth or dry white wine
- 1 cup frozen peas, defrosted
- ½ cup cream
- salt and freshly ground black pepper

1. Add enough water to a pot and bring to the boil. Add the *eisbein* and bring back to the boil. Skim off any scum that rises to the surface.
2. Add the remaining ingredients to the pot and reduce to a slow simmer. The water must just bubble.
3. Cook the *eisbein* for 1 ½ to 2 hours, until the meat is tender and almost falling off the bone. Occasionally skim off any scum that rises.
4. To prepare the pea puree: add the butter to a saucepan on medium heat. Fry the bacon until crisp. Remove with a slotted spoon.
5. Add the shallot, carrot and celery and sauté for about 5 minutes, or until softened. Add the peas, marjoram and thyme.
6. Pour in the vermouth or wine and deglaze the pan. Cook until almost all the liquid has evaporated. If the vegetables are not yet tender, add a little of the *eisbein* water and cook a little longer.

7. Add half the cream to the pea mixture and puree in a countertop blender until smooth. Return to the pot. Alternatively puree in the saucepan using a hand stick blender.
8. Bring the pea puree back to a simmer and stir in the remaining cream, or until you have the desired consistency. The pea puree must not be too thin. Season to taste with salt and freshly ground black pepper.
9. Place an *eisbein* on each plate. Add a good dollop of pea puree sprinkled with crispy bacon and serve with sauerkraut and boiled parsley potatoes.

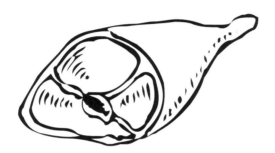

Hunter's Cutlet
Jägerschnitzel

Preparation time: **20 min**
Cooking time: **30 min**

Ingredients:
4 Servings

- 1 tbsp butter
- 3 rashers streaky bacon, diced
- 1 small onion, diced
- 16 oz mushrooms, thickly sliced
- ¼ cup red wine
- ½ cup beef stock
- 1 ½ tsp fresh thyme or ½ tsp dried thyme
- 1 bay leaf
- 1 small bunch parsley, chopped (reserve some for garnish)
- ½ cup cream
- 8 de-boned pork loin cutlets, trimmed of any fat
- Fresh ground or fine sea salt, to taste
- freshly ground black pepper, to taste
- all-purpose flour for dusting cutlets
- 3 eggs, beaten
- breadcrumbs
- ½ cup lard or clarified butter (alternatively use ½ butter & ½ vegetable oil)

---

1. Add the butter to a saucepan on medium heat. When melted add the bacon and onions and fry for about 2 minutes, or until the onions have softened. Add the mushrooms and cook for a further 3 minutes.
2. Add the red wine, beef stock, thyme, bay leaf, parsley, cream and black pepper to taste. Gently simmer until the sauce has reduced by half, or has thickened to a desired consistency. Taste and add salt and pepper, if desired. Remove the bay leaf, cover with a lid and keep warm.
3. Place a slice of pork cutlet between 2 sheets of plastic wrap and pound with a meat mallet, or a rolling pin, until about a ¼ inch thick. Repeat with remaining cutlets.
4. Season the pork cutlets on both sides with salt and black pepper to taste.

5. Add the flour, beaten eggs and breadcrumbs to separate large bowls or plates.
6. Dust a cutlet on both sides with flour, shaking off the excess. Dip into the beaten egg, ensuring you cover both sides well. Coat with breadcrumbs, gently pressing the crumbs to ensure they stick if necessary. Repeat with remaining cutlets.
7. Heat the lard or butter in a large, heavy-bottomed skillet or frying pan on medium-high heat.
8. Fry the cutlets until golden brown on both sides. Do this in batches so as not to overcrowd the pan – this will drop the temperature and the cutlets will become greasy. Remove the cutlets to paper towel to remove excess fat.
9. To serve: pour the sauce over a ⅓ of the cutlet, sprinkle with parsley and serve with a lemon wedge or slices.

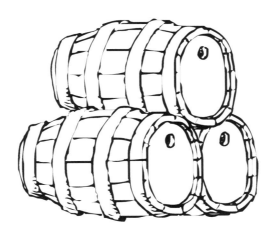

Marinated Beef Pot Roast
Sauerbraten

Preparation time: **30 min + 48 - 72 h marinating**
Cooking time: **2 h**

Ingredients:
6 Servings

- 2 cups medium-bodied red wine
- 1 cup red wine vinegar
- 1 cup water, or as needed
- 2 large onions, diced
- 2 large carrots, diced
- 3 sticks celery, diced
- 12 black peppercorns
- 8 juniper berries, crushed
- 4 bay leaves
- 3 tbsp Sauerbraten spice mix
- 3 lbs. bottom round roast
- 1 tbsp lard (schmaltz) or vegetable oil
- 12 gingersnap cookies (lebkuchen), crumbed (alternatively use pumpernickel)
- 2 thin slices pumpernickel, crumbed (alternative to gingersnap cookies)
- ⅓ cup raisins (optional)
- 3 tbsp red wine
- ½ cup heavy cream

---

1. Bring the wine to the boil in a large Dutch oven or oven-proof casserole pot to cook off the alcohol. Remove from the heat and add the all the remaining ingredients except the beef and lard. Allow to cool completely.
2. Add the beef to a large glass or ceramic bowl and pour over the marinade. The marinade must cover the beef. Add more water or wine if necessary. Cover tightly with plastic wrap and marinate in the fridge for 2 to 3 days. Turn the beef over at least twice a day.
3. Remove the beef from the marinade and pat dry with kitchen paper. Season with salt and pepper.
4. Add the lard or oil to the Dutch oven on high heat. Sear the beef in the hot fat until nicely browned all over.
5. Remove the beef from the pot and add the marinade. Stir and scrap off all the caramelized 'bits' have stuck to the bottom of the pot. Remove from the heat and return the beef to the pot.
6. Place the pot in an oven pre-heated to 350° F and cook for 2 hours.
7. Turn the beef every 30 minutes. Add more water if necessary so that the beef is covered ½ way up.

8. Remove the beef to a warm serving platter, cover with aluminum foil and set aside in a warm place.
9. Strain the marinade and return to a clean saucepan. Leave for a few minutes for the fat to rise to the surface and then skim off. Alternatively use a fat separator jug to remove the excess fat.
10. Bring the sauce to the boil and then reduce to a simmer. Taste, and add salt and pepper if needed. Add the gingersnaps or pumpernickel and stir until dissolved into the sauce. Optional: strain the sauce again to remove any lumps.
11. Add the (optional) raisins, 3 tablespoons of red wine and the cream, and simmer until the sauce has thickened.
12. Slice the beef and pour over the sauce.

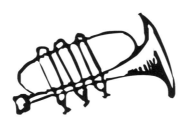

Roasted Pork Knuckle
Schweinshaxe

Preparation time: **15 min**
Cooking time: **3 h**

Ingredients:

2 Servings

- 1 ½ tsp caraway seeds
- 3 cloves
- 4 bay leaves
- 2 tbsp parsley (including stems), chopped
- 1 tsp freshly ground black pepper
- 1 tsp sea salt
- 1 large onion, diced
- 1 carrot, diced
- 1 stick celery, diced
- 4 cloves garlic, crushed
- 1 ½ cups (12 oz) bock beer (dark lager)
- 1 ½ cups water
- 2 fresh pork knuckles

---

1. Add all the ingredients, except the pork knuckles, to a large Dutch oven, or large pot with a lid, and bring to the boil.
2. Add the pork knuckles and bring back to the boil. Skim off any scum that rises to the surface.
3. Reduce the heat to medium. It should be just a gentle boil.
4. Place the lid on and cook for 1 hour. Turn the knuckles every 15 minutes or so, and skim off any scum that has risen. If needed add a little extra water.
5. Pre-heat the oven to 375° F
6. Take the knuckles out, and using a sharp knife, score the skin several times, especially the fatty parts.
7. Place on a rack in a roasting pan with the bone sticking up (resting on thickest part).
8. Remove the bay leaves from the cooking liquid and use a hand stick blender to blend the liquid.
9. Pour the blended cooking liquid into the roasting pan.
10. Roast the knuckles for about 2 hours, or until nice a crispy and browned. Baste with pan juices from time to time.
11. The pan juices can be used as a base for a sauce after skimming off excess fat.
12. Place the knuckle on a plate with the bone pointing up and serve with your choice of red cabbage, sauerkraut, potatoes, mashed potato and mustard.

Sausage with Apple-Sauerkraut
Wurst mit Apfel-Sauerkraut

Preparation time: **10 min**

Cooking time: **1 h**

Ingredients:

4 Servings

- 2 tbsp olive oil or lard
- 4 oz slab smoked bacon, sliced into ½ inch pieces
- 1 large red onion, chopped
- ½ cup Riesling (alternatively use bock-style beer)
- 1 large Golden Delicious apple, peeled, cored, ½ inch dice
- 4 bay leaves, fresh preferably
- 8 juniper berries, crushed
- ½ tsp caraway seeds (optional)
- ½ tsp freshly ground black pepper
- 1 tsp sugar, or to taste
- ½ cup water
- 3 cups (16 oz) sauerkraut, drained and squeezed dry
- salt, to taste
- ½ cup frozen peas, defrosted (optional)
- 8 bockwurst, or other smoked German sausage
- 2 tbsp parsley, chopped

1. Heat 1 tablespoon of olive oil or lard in a skillet and fry the bacon until crisp. Remove the bacon and set aside.
2. Reduce the heat to low and add the onions to the same pan and gently cook until softened, about 10 minutes.
3. Add the wine, apple, bay leaves, juniper berries, caraway seeds, pepper, sugar and salt to the onions, bring to the boil and cook on medium high heat for 3 minutes. Note: the sauerkraut is salty so be careful with the amount of salt added. You can always add more later.
4. Add the water and sauerkraut. Reduce the heat to low and cook for 30 minutes, or until the apples are tender.
5. Whilst the sauerkraut is cooking prepare the sausages. Make several small cuts on each side of the sausages.
6. Heat the remaining tablespoon of olive oil or lard in a large skillet. Fry the sausages on medium heat, turning a few times, until heated through and nicely browned.
7. Taste the sauerkraut and season with salt and pepper if desired.
8. Optional: stir the peas into the sauerkraut.
9. Add the sausages to the sauerkraut and cook for 3 minutes.
10. Spoon the sauerkraut onto a warm serving plate, place the sausages on top and sprinkle over the bacon and chopped parsley.

35

Boiled Beef with Horseradish Sauce
Tafelspitz mit Meerrettichsoße

Preparation time: **30 min**

Cooking time: **2 h 20 min (plus 10 min resting time)**

Ingredients:

4 Servings

- 6 ⅓ pt. water
- ½ medium bunch flat leaf (Italian) parsley, chopped
- 3 bay leaves
- 12 black peppercorns
- 1 tsp ground allspice
- 1 tbsp coarse sea (kosher) salt, or to taste
- 3 - 3 ½ lbs. top round beef
- 1 medium celeriac, sliced into ¼-inch batons
- 3 large onions, sliced
- 3 large carrots, halved and sliced into ¼-inch batons
- 2 medium leeks, halved and sliced lengthways
- ½ stick (2 oz) butter
- 5 tbsp all-purpose flour
- 2 cups reserved broth from Tafelspitz
- ½ cup fresh horseradish, peeled and grated
- ¾ cup heavy cream
- 1 ½ tsp fresh lemon juice
- 1 - 1 ½ tsp sugar, or to taste
- salt, to taste
- ¼ cup reserved broth from the Tafelspitz
- chopped parsley for garnish

1. Add the water, parsley, bay leaves, peppercorns, allspice and salt to a large Dutch oven and bring to the boil.
2. Add the beef to the water, reduce to simmer, place the lid on and cook for 2 hours, or until tender. Adjust the heat so that the water just bubbles. Occasionally skim off any scum that rises.
3. Add the celeriac, onions, carrots and leeks to the pot and cook for a further 20 minutes, with the lid on.
4. Remove the beef to a warm serving platter and cover with aluminum foil. Set aside for at least 10 minutes to rest whilst you prepare the horseradish sauce.
5. Strain the broth and reserve 2 cups for the horseradish sauce and ¼ cup for serving. Add the vegetables back to the pot, place the lid on and keep warm.
6. Melt the butter in a saucepan on medium heat. Add the flour and stir into the butter until well combined. Cook for a further 2 – 3 minutes, stirring constantly, until lightly browned.

37

7. Gradually add the reserved 2 cups of broth whisking constantly until you have a smooth sauce with no lumps. Add the cream and bring to the boil. Reduce the heat to low, add the horseradish and cook for a further 5 minutes, stirring occasionally.
8. Season to taste with lemon juice, sugar and salt.
9. Slice the beef on the serving platter, add the vegetables on top and drizzle over the ¼ cup of reserved broth.
10. Garnish with a sprinkling of parsley and serve with the horseradish sauce.

Pan-Fried Beef Steaks with Onions
Zwiebelrostbraten

Preparation time: **10 min**
Cooking time: **30 min**

Ingredients:
2 Servings

- 4 onions, sliced and separated into rings
- 1 tsp paprika
- 2 tbsp butter
- 2 (7 oz) sirloin or rib-eye steaks, ¼ inch thick
- 2 tbsp Dijon mustard
- 2 tbsp canola oil
- 1 tbsp tomato paste
- 1 tbsp all-purpose flour
- ⅓ cup red wine
- ¾ cup beef broth
- ¼ cup light cream
- salt, freshly ground black pepper and paprika, to taste

1. Season the onion rings with paprika and salt to taste. Heat the butter in a frying pan on medium heat. Fry the onions until softened and golden brown, about 10 minutes. Set aside.
2. If the steaks are too thick, place between 2 sheets of plastic wrap and flatten with a meat mallet or rolling pin. Brush both sides of the steaks with mustard.
3. Heat the oil in a heavy-bottomed skillet on high heat. Fry the steaks for about 2 minutes on each side. Remove from the pan and season with salt and black pepper to taste.
4. Reduce the heat to medium and stir the flour into the remaining oil in the pan. Cook for 1 minute, stirring constantly. Deglaze the pan with red wine, ensuring you scrape off any bits stuck to the pan.
5. Add the beef broth and simmer for about 10 minutes, or until reduced by half. Add the cream and simmer for another 2 – 3 minutes, or until thickened. Season to taste with salt, pepper and paprika.
6. Re-heat the onions.
7. Re-heat the steaks in the sauce for a minute or two, turning once.
8. To serve pour the sauce over the steaks and top with fried onions.

Brandenburg Braised Lamb
Brandenburger Lammfleisch

Preparation time: **15 min**

Cooking time: **1 h 20 min**

Ingredients:

4 - 6 Servings

- 2 – 3 tbsp lard or canola oil
- salt and black pepper, to taste
- all-purpose flour, for dusting lamb
- 2 lbs. lamb shoulder, cut into 1½" cubes (trimmed of excess fat)
- ½ cup red wine
- 2 onions, diced
- 2 cups lamb or chicken stock
- 1 tsp dried marjoram
- 1 ½ lbs. fresh green beans, top & tailed & halved
- 1 lb. potatoes, peeled and diced
- 1 tbsp fresh summer savory, chopped (alt. use ½ thyme & ½ sage)

1. Heat 1 tablespoon lard in a large Dutch oven, or heavy-bottomed pot, on high heat.
2. Season the lamb with salt and pepper, and coat with a light dusting of flour.
3. Sear the meat, in batches, until well browned. Add extra lard as needed. Set aside.
4. Deglaze the pot with red wine, scraping up all the bits stuck to the bottom. Pour the deglaze liquid into the stock.
5. Add a tablespoon of lard to the pot on medium heat. Sauté the onions until softened, about 5 minutes.
6. Add the lamb, stock and marjoram to the pot. Cover with a lid and gently simmer for about one hour.
7. Add the beans and potatoes. Taste the liquid and season with salt and pepper. Simmer for another 20 minutes, or until the potatoes are tender.
8. Taste again and add salt and pepper if desired.
9. Serve garnished with a sprinkling of savory.

Classic Beef Goulash
Klassisches Gulasch

Preparation time: **15 min**
Cooking time: **2 h 30 min**

Ingredients:
6 – 8 Servings

- 3.5 oz lard (approx. ½ cup)
- 7 large onions, sliced
- 2 large cloves garlic, minced
- 1 tbsp all-purpose flour
- 1 cup red wine
- 1 ½ cups beef stock
- 1 ½ cups water
- 1 tbsp tomato paste
- 3 tbsp sweet paprika
- 1 tbsp hot paprika
- 2 tsp caraway seeds, ground
- ¼ tsp allspice
- 1 tbsp marjoram
- 1 tsp lemon zest, finely chopped
- 1 tsp brown sugar
- 1 ½ tsp kosher salt, or to taste
- 1 tsp freshly ground black pepper
- 2 tbsp parsley, chopped
- 3 ½ lbs. beef shin, cut into 1inch pieces

1. Melt lard in a large pot with a lid, on medium high heat.
2. Brown the beef on all sides. Do this in batches so as not to overcrowd the pot. Remove and set aside.
3. Reduce the heat to medium and add the onions. Fry until softened and golden brown, about 8 to 10 minutes.
4. Add the garlic and cook for another minute. Stir in the flour.
5. Pour in the wine and deglaze the pot. Add the stock and water.
6. Stir in the tomato paste, paprika, caraway seeds, allspice, marjoram, lemon zest, sugar, salt, pepper and half the parsley. Bring to the boil.
7. Add the beef and reduce to a gentle simmer. Place the lid on and cook for 2 ½ hours, or until the meat is tender.
8. Stir the pot regularly. If needed add some more water.
9. Remove the meat from the pot to a warm serving plate.
10. Taste the sauce and adjust seasoning with salt and pepper if desired.
11. If necessary raise the heat and cook the sauce until thickened.
12. Pour the sauce over the beef and sprinkle with the remaining parsley.
13. Serve with your choice of potatoes, flat noodles (e.g. tagliatelle), spätzle, rice or dumplings.

Leberkäse

Leberkäse

Preparation time: **45 min**
Cooking time: **1 h 30 min**

Ingredients:
6 Servings
- 1 lb. pork shoulder, diced
- 1 lb. rindless pork belly, diced
- 1 ½ tbsp kosher salt
- ¾ tsp white pepper, or to taste
- 1 tsp dried marjoram
- 1 tsp dried thyme
- ½ tsp ground cinnamon
- ½ tsp ground nutmeg
- ½ tsp ground ginger
- 10 oz ice cubes
- 1 onion, finely grated
- 5 rashers smoked bacon, finely diced (optional)
- butter for greasing pan

1. Pre-heat the oven to 320° F.
2. Place the diced meat in the freezer for 30 minutes.
3. Mix the herbs and spices together.
4. Remove the meat from the freezer.
5. Add the meat, salt, pepper, herbs and spices to a food processor bowl, with the blade fitted.
6. Process the meat, adding cubes of ice, until you have a smooth, well-blended paste.
7. Remove the meat from the processor to a bowl. Add the onion and (optional) bacon, and mix together until thoroughly combined with the meat.
8. Butter a suitable loaf pan with butter.
9. Add the meat paste to the loaf tin. Firmly tap the loaf tin on a counter a few times to settle the meat into the pan and remove any air-pockets. Smooth the top using a spatula.
10. Use a sharp knife to slash a diamond-pattern, about ¼-inch deep, on the top of the meatloaf.
11. Bake on the center rack of the oven for 90 minutes, or until set and nicely browned on top. If necessary brown for 5 minutes under the oven grill.

Munich Style Schnitzel
Münchner Schnitzel

Preparation time: **15 min**
Cooking time: **12 min**

Ingredients:
4 Servings

- veal scaloppini, 5 – 6 oz each,
- freshly ground sea salt, to taste
- freshly ground black pepper, to taste
- tbsp sweet German mustard, or Dijon mustard
- tbsp creamed horseradish, or to taste (alternatively use fresh grated)
- all-purpose flour for dusting scaloppini
- eggs, beaten
- breadcrumbs
- ½ cup lard or clarified butter (alternatively use ½ butter & ½ canola oil)
- lemon wedges

1. The veal scaloppini should be about ½ inch thick. To flatten, place a slice of scaloppini between 2 sheets of plastic wrap and pound with a meat mallet, or a rolling pin, until about a ½ inch thick. Repeat with remaining scaloppini.
2. Season the veal on both sides with salt and black pepper, to taste.
3. Spread one side with mustard and the other side with horseradish.
4. Alternatively, if using fresh grated horseradish: mix the horseradish with the mustard. Spread the mixture on both sides of the scaloppini.
5. Add the flour, beaten eggs and breadcrumbs to separate large bowls or plates.
6. Dust a scaloppini on both sides with flour, shaking off the excess.
7. Dip into the beaten egg, ensuring you cover both sides well.
8. Coat with breadcrumbs. Gently press the breadcrumbs in to ensure they stick, if necessary. Repeat with remaining scaloppini.
9. Heat the lard or butter in a large, heavy-bottomed skillet or frying pan on medium-high heat.
10. Fry the scaloppini until golden brown on both sides. Do this in batches so as not to overcrowd the pan – this will drop the temperature and the scaloppini will become greasy.
11. Remove the scaloppini to paper towel to drain excess fat.
12. Serve with lemon wedges.

Pichelsteiner One-pot Meat Stew
Pichelsteiner Eintopf

Preparation time: **30 min**

Cooking time: **1 h 30 min**

Ingredients:

6 Servings

- 4 tbsp lard or canola oil
- ½ lb. boneless beef chuck, cut into 1-inch cubes
- ½ lb. boneless pork shoulder, cut into 1-inch cubes
- ½ lb. boneless lamb shoulder or boneless veal neck, cut into 1-inch cubes
- ¼ lb. pork belly, cut into 1-inch cubes
- 1 large onion, diced
- 1 leek, cut into ½" pieces
- 3 carrots, peeled and cut into ¾" pieces
- 1 small celeriac (celery root), ½" dice
- 1 small savoy cabbage, coarsely chopped
- 1 large stick celery, diced
- 2 parsnips, peeled and diced
- 1 kohlrabi, peeled and diced
- 3 medium potatoes, peeled and cut into ½" dice
- 4 pts. beef stock
- 1 tsp ground caraway
- 1 tbsp paprika
- 1 tsp marjoram
- 1 bunch parsley, chopped (including stems)
- salt and black pepper, to taste

1. Heat 2 tablespoons of lard in a large Dutch oven or pot on high heat. Sear all the meats, in batches, until well browned. Set aside.
2. Reduce the heat to medium and deglaze the pot with a little beef stock if necessary. Add deglaze liquid back to stock.
3. Add a tbsp. of lard to the pot and sauté the onion and leek for 5 minutes. Set aside
4. Add the remaining lard to the pot and sauté the remaining vegetables, excluding the potato, for 5 minutes. If necessary do this in batches. Set aside.
5. Stir the caraway, paprika, marjoram and parsley into the beef stock.
6. Add the ingredients to the pot in 2 layers, seasoning each layer well with salt and pepper.
7. First add a layer of meat, then the onion, then the vegetables and finally a layer of potatoes. Repeat.
8. Pour over the beef stock and bring to the boil over high heat.

9. Reduce the heat to lowest and cover with the lid. Gently simmer for 1 ½ hours. Do not stir.
10. Alternatively cook for 1 ½ - 2 hours in the oven set to 350° F.

Stuffed Beef Rolls
Rinderrouladen

Preparation time: **30 min**

Cooking time: **1 h 50 min**

Ingredients:

4 Servings

- 3 tbsp canola oil
- 2 sweet onions, halved and sliced
- 4 slices top round, about 8" long x 4" wide & ¼" thick (about 1 ½lbs)
- 1 tsp paprika
- salt and freshly ground black pepper, to taste
- 2 tbsp German (or Dijon) mustard
- 8 rashers smoked bacon
- 2 dill pickles, cut lengthways into ¼'s
- ¼ cup canola oil

For the gravy

- ¼ cup red wine
- 2 cups beef stock
- 1 tsp tomato paste
- 1 tsp German (or Dijon) mustard
- ¼ tsp paprika
- 2 tbsp parsley, chopped
- 2 tbsp cornstarch
- 2 tbsp water
- salt and pepper to taste

1. Heat 3 tablespoons canola oil in a large Dutch oven or large heavy-bottom pot with a lid. Fry the onions until softened. Remove from the pot and set aside to cool.
2. Lay the slices of beef on a cutting board and season with paprika, salt and pepper, and spread with mustard.
3. Lay two bacon rashers onto each slice of beef, trimming any bits that extend over the edges. Evenly sprinkle over the onions.
4. Place a pickle slice, crossways, on the widest end of the short side. It should be about an inch from the edge.
5. Take the widest end, fold over the pickle and start rolling until completely rolled up.
6. Firmly tie each roulade with string in 2 or 3 places. Trim any bits of pickle that extend over the edges. Repeat with remaining slices.
7. Heat the remaining ¼ cup of oil in the Dutch oven on high heat. Sear the rouladen, in batches, until well browned all over.
8. Reduce the heat to medium and deglaze the pot with red wine. Add the stock, tomato paste, mustard, paprika and parsley, and stir to combine. Bring to the boil.

9. Reduce the heat to low and add the rouladen. Place the lid on and cook for 1 ½ hours, or until tender. Turn the rouladen over a few times during cooking.
10. Remove the rouladen to a warm serving plate and remove the string. Cover loosely with aluminum foil.
11. Dissolve the cornstarch with the water. Stir into the sauce and bring to the boil, stirring constantly, until thickened. Taste and season with salt and pepper if desired.
12. Pour the sauce over the rouladen and sprinkle with parsley if desired.

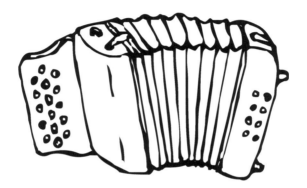

Onion Tart
Zwiebelkuchen

Preparation time: **30 min + 1 h dough proving time**
Cooking time: **40 min**

Ingredients:
6 Servings
For the dough
- 3 cups all-purpose flour
- 1 tsp salt
- 1 ½ tsp instant yeast
- 1 ½ cups water, lukewarm
- butter for greasing springform pan

For the filling
- 5 white onions, peeled, halved and sliced
- 3 tbsp canola oil
- ½ cup cream
- ¼ cup crème fraiche or sour cream
- ½ tsp salt, or to taste
- 1 large egg, beaten
- 1 large egg yolk, beaten together with whole egg
- ¼ tsp ground nutmeg
- 1 tsp caraway seeds, or to taste
- salt and freshly ground black pepper, to taste
- 3 – 4 slices smoked bacon (about 3 tbsp crumbled bacon)

1. Pre-heat the oven to 350° F.
2. Sift the flour, salt and yeast into a mixing bowl. Add the water and mix until you have a smooth and elastic dough.
3. Form the dough into a ball and oil the surface. Cover the bowl with a dish cloth and leave to rise in a warm place for an hour.
4. Add half the oil to a large skillet or frying pan on medium heat. Add the onions and cook for 15 to 20 minutes, or until the onions are soft and lightly browned. Add more oil to the skillet as necessary. Remove from the heat and set aside.
5. Add a little oil to the pan and fry the bacon until very crispy. Allow to cool and then crumble into bits. Mix with the cooked onions.
6. Mix together, in a clean bowl, the cream, crème fraiche, eggs, nutmeg, and salt and pepper to taste.
7. Grease an 11-inch springform pan with butter. Alternatively use and 11 x 13-inch baking pan with at least 1½-inch sides.
8. Press the dough evenly into the pan ensuring that you form 1½-inch sides.
9. Spread the onion and bacon mixture evenly on the dough. Pour the cream mixture over the onions, titling the pan to spread evenly.

10. Sprinkle over the caraway seeds.
11. Bake on the center shelf of the pre-heated oven for 40 to 45 minutes, or until set and the top is golden brown. If the dough doesn't seem crispy enough cover loosely with aluminum foil and bake for a further 5 minutes.
12. Remove from the oven and set aside for 5 minutes before removing from the springform pan.

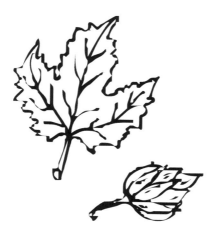

Egg Noodles with Bacon & Cheese
Spätzle mit Speck und Käse

Preparation time: **30 min**

Cooking time: **25 min**

Ingredients:

6 Servings

For the spaetzle

- cups all-purpose flour
- ¼ tsp freshly ground nutmeg
- ½ tsp salt, or to taste
- large free-range eggs, beaten
- 1 ¼ cups whole milk, or as needed (or water for a less-rich spaetzle)

For the sauce

- 1 onion, thinly sliced
- 2 tbsp butter
- 6 - 8 slices smoked bacon, diced
- 7 oz good quality smoked German cheese or Emmental, grated
- oz smoked Black Forest ham
- 2 cups heavy cream
- 3 tbsp chives, chopped

1. Sift the flour, nutmeg and salt together and add to the bowl of a stand mixer with a dough hook fitted.
2. Add the eggs and milk. Mix the dough on medium speed for about 15 minutes, until you have a smooth, loose dough. Pull the dough with a wooden spoon. Holes should appear. If the dough is too wet or too stiff, add extra flour or milk, as needed, and knead a little longer.
3. Let the dough rest for 30 – 60 minutes.
4. Bring a large pot of well-salted boiling water to a simmering boil.
5. Spaetzle maker method: fill the maker with dough and press to squeeze the noodles out into the simmering water. Simmer the noodles for 2 to 3 minutes, or until they float to the surface. Remove the noodles with a slotted spoon and place in a bowl of cold water to cool before draining in a colander. Repeat until all the dough has been used.
6. Colander method: hold a large-holed colander over the pot of simmering water, with the colander at least 3 – 4 inches above the surface of the water. Dip the colander into the simmering water to moisten. Add a ladle of dough to the colander and press through using a large spoon or dough scraper (also dipped into the simmering water – it helps prevent the dough sticking). Simmer the noodles for 2 to 3 minutes, or until they float to the surface. Remove

the noodles with a slotted spoon and place in a bowl of cold water to cool before draining in a colander. Repeat, frequently dipping the scraper into the water, until all the dough has been used.

7. Spaetzle board method (wood or metal board): dip the board into the simmering water to moisten. A straight-edged metal spatula or knife, or a straight-edged plastic dough scraper is needed to scrape the dough into the water. Dip the board into the simmering water, add a ladle of dough and spread thinly with a moistened spatula. Working as quickly as possible, scrape thin slices of dough off the board into the simmering water. Dip the spatula and the end of the board regularly into the simmering water. Moistening helps with scraping the dough off the board. Simmer the noodles for 2 to 3 minutes, or until they float to the surface. Remove the noodles with a slotted spoon and place in a bowl of cold water to cool before draining in a colander. Repeat until all the dough has been used.

8. Pre-heat the oven to 350° F.

9. Add the spaetzle to a baking dish.

10. Heat the butter in a skillet and sauté the onions and bacon for 8 minutes, until the onions are softened. Stir in the chives.

11. Heat the cream in a saucepan on medium heat. Season with salt and freshly ground black pepper. Be cautious with the salt as the bacon and ham are salty. Add the cheese (reserve some for the top) and stir until melted and incorporated. Stir in the ham. Pour over the spaetzle and stir to mix well.

12. Scatter over the fried onion and bacon mixture, and the reserved cheese.

13. Bake for 15 – 20 minutes, or until hot and the top is bubbly and nicely browned.

Meat Balls in White Sauce with Capers
Königsberger Klopse

Preparation time: **30 min**

Cooking time: **25 min**

Ingredients:

4 Servings

For the dumplings

- 2 stale bread rolls
- ½ cup milk
- 1 tbsp canola oil
- 1 medium onion, halved
- 1 white onion, diced
- 3 anchovy fillets (optional)
- 9 oz. ground chicken or turkey
- 9 oz. ground pork
- 3 medium eggs, beaten
- 3 tbsp capers, chopped
- 1 tbsp whole grain mustard
- 1 cup parsley, chopped
- 1 tbsp kosher salt, or to taste
- freshly ground black pepper, to taste
- 4 ½ cups chicken broth
- 2 cloves
- 3 bay leaves

For the caper cream sauce

- 3 tbsp butter
- 2 tbsp all-purpose flour
- ½ cup white wine
- ½ cream (or half-and-half for a less rich sauce)
- 1 – 2 cups cooking broth from dumplings, or as needed
- 2 tbsp capers
- pinch of ground nutmeg
- 1 tsp fresh lemon juice, or to taste (optional)
- salt and black pepper, to taste
- chopped parsley for garnish

1. Soak the bread rolls in milk for about 10 minutes. Squeeze the excess milk from the bread after soaking and rub to crumble.
2. Brush the cut surfaces of the halved onion with oil. The onion does not need to be peeled. Cut the onion in half through the middle and not the root end. Sear the cut surfaces in a hot skillet or frying pan until well browned, but not burnt. Set aside.
3.   Reduce the heat to medium and sauté the diced onions in the remaining oil until softened, about 8 minutes. Be careful not to brown

the onions as it will color the cream sauce. Add the anchovy fillets and gently cook, stirring to break them up and help them dissolve into the onions, about 3 minutes.

4. Add the soaked bread crumbs, cooked onions, ground chicken, ground pork, eggs, capers, mustard, parsley, salt and pepper to a large bowl. Use your hand to mix the ingredients together until thoroughly combined. Use damp hands to firmly form the meat mixture into 8 balls.

5. Add the chicken broth, cloves, bay leaves and the browned onion halves to a large pot and bring to the boil. Reduce to a gentle simmer and add the dumplings. Poach for 10 – 12 minutes.

6. Melt the butter in a saucepan on medium heat. Stir in the flour, being careful not to brown the flour. When well combined stir in the white wine. Cook until reduced by half.

7. Stir in the cream and 1 cup of broth, constantly stirring. As the sauce starts to thicken gradually add the second cup of broth until the sauce is the desired thickness, about the consistency of cream. Add the capers, nutmeg and season to taste with salt, pepper and lemon juice.

8. Remove the dumplings from the broth with a slotted spoon and add to the cream sauce. Simmer gently for 3 minutes in the sauce.

9. Serve sprinkled with parsley.

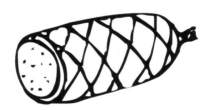

Alsatian Schnitzel
Elsässer Schnitzel

Preparation time: **20 min**
Cooking time: **10 min**

Ingredients:
4 Servings

- 8 slices pork tenderloin, about ½" thick (about 1 ½ lbs.)
- salt and black pepper, to taste
- ground nutmeg, to taste
- 1 clove garlic, peeled and halved
- 2 tbsp canola oil
- 1 cup sour cream or crème fraiche
- 1 large onion, sliced into rings
- 5 oz smoked raw pickled ham or smoked slab bacon, diced into ¼" cubes
- ½ cup Gruyère cheese, grated
- Fresh parsley or chives for garnish, chopped

1. I f necessary flatten the pork tenderloin between 2 pieces of plastic wrap using a meat mallet or rolling pin.
2. Pre-heat the oven to 400° F.
3. Rub the base and sides of a porcelain or earthenware baking dish with the garlic.
4. Season both sides of the pork with salt, pepper and nutmeg.
5. Heat the oil in a heavy-bottomed skillet or frying pan on high heat. Sear the pork slices for half a minute on each side.
6. Place the seared pork into the baking dish and cover with cream.
7. Scatter over the onion rings and the ham (or bacon).
8. Sprinkle with cheese.
9. Bake in the pre-heated oven for 10 – 15 minutes, or until the ham is cooked and the cheese bubbly and nicely browned.
10. Garnish with parsley or chives and serve.

Desserts

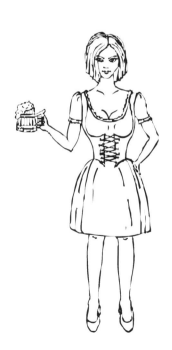

Apple Strudel

Apfelstrudel

Preparation time: **30 min**
Cooking time: **35 min**

Ingredients:
6 Servings

- 3 tbsp butter
- 1 cup fresh white breadcrumbs
- 1 tsp cinnamon powder
- ⅓ cup sliced toasted almonds
- ½ cup golden sultanas
- ½ cup raisins
- 1 ½ lbs. Granny Smith, Pink Lady or other cooking apples
- 2 tbsp fresh lemon juice
- 1 tbsp lemon zest, finely grated
- 2 tbsp light rum
- ½ cup sugar
- 8 sheets phyllo pastry
- ½ stick (4 oz.) butter, melted
- confectioner's sugar for dusting

1. Pre-heat the oven to 375° F. Melt 3 tbsp butter in a frying pan. Add the breadcrumbs and cook over medium heat until toasted and golden brown. Stir in the cinnamon and almonds.
2. Peel, core and halve the apples. Thinly slice and add to a large bowl. Toss together with lemon juice, lemon zest, rum and sugar.
3. Place a sheet of greaseproof kitchen paper on a counter top.
4. Lay a sheet of phyllo over and brush with melted butter. Evenly sprinkle over some of the breadcrumb mixture. Lay another sheet of phyllo over, brush with butter and sprinkle with breadcrumb mixture. Repeat with remaining sheets of phyllo.
5. Turn the phyllo sheets so that a long side faces you.
6. Spoon the apple mixture evenly across the phyllo, leaving a 1-inch border on both sides. Spread the apple mixture until it is about 2 inches from the bottom edge. Sprinkle over leftover breadcrumb mix.
7. Fold the side edges over and then fold the bottom edge over. Ensure the edges are well brushed with butter.
8. Roll the strudel into a fat sausage. Squeeze the edges to seal.
9. Line a baking tray with baking paper. Slide the strudel onto the tray, with the seam side down. Brush with leftover melted butter.
10. Place on the center rack of the oven and bake for 30 to 35 minutes, or until nicely browned and crisp.
11. Cool on a wire rack for 10 minutes. Dust with confectioner's sugar and serve with vanilla sauce, whipped cream or ice cream.

Red Berry Fruit Compote
Rote Grütze

Preparation time: **30 min**
Cooking time: **25 min**

Ingredients:

6 Servings

- 3 tbsp sugar, or to taste
- ¾ cup cranberry or red grape juice
- 2 - 3 tbsp Cassis, Kirschwasser or berry liqueur of choice
- ⅓ cup red wine
- ½ tsp vanilla extract
- ½ tsp cinnamon powder
- 3 tbsp arrowroot or cornstarch, or as needed
- 1 lb. mixed berries (raspberries, strawberries, redcurrants, blackberries, blueberries)
- 1 cup (about 5 oz) pitted Morello cherries
- 2 tbsp dark or milk chocolate, grated
- fresh mint leaves for garnish

For the vanilla sauce

- ½ cup whole milk
- ⅓ cup cream
- 1 vanilla bean, split lengthways or 1 tsp vanilla extract
- 2 tbsp sugar, or to taste
- 2 egg yolks, beaten

1. Add the sugar, fruit juice, Cassis and red wine to a pot on medium heat. Bring to the boil and stir to dissolve the sugar. Reduce to a simmer and stir in the vanilla and cinnamon.
2. Dissolve the arrowroot in 3 tablespoons of cold water. Slowly pour into the hot liquid, stirring constantly, until the liquid has thickened. Use more diluted arrowroot if the liquid is too runny, or add more fruit juice if too thick.
3. Add the berries to the liquid, reserve a cup of berries for garnishing. Stir to combine and cook for 3 min, or until berries have just softened.
4. Pour the compote into serving cups or bowls and refrigerate whilst preparing the vanilla sauce.
5. Add the milk, cream, vanilla and sugar to a saucepan and bring to almost boiling. Reduce the heat to medium low.
6. Remove from the heat and whisk in the egg yolks. Return to the heat and cook until thickened, stirring constantly. Remove from the heat and strain through a sieve to remove any lumps and the vanilla pod. Set aside to cool.
7. To serve pour vanilla sauce over the compote, sprinkle with grated chocolate and garnish with the reserved berries and mint leaves.

Black Forest Gateau
Schwarzwälder Kirschtorte

Preparation time: **30 min**

Cooking time: **50 min**

Ingredients:

8-10 Servings

For the sponge

- 7 oz unsalted butter, softened
- 1 cup superfine sugar
- 6 large free-range eggs, separated
- 1 cup (4.5 oz) all-purpose flour
- 1 ½ tsp baking powder
- ½ tsp kosher salt
- 10 tbsp (2.5 oz) cocoa powder
- 3 tbsp whole milk

For the filling & topping

- 3 tbsp Kirschwasser
- 4 tbsp cherry jam, preferably Morello or dark cherry
- 4 cups (32 fl. oz) heavy cream, whipped
- 1 tsp vanilla extract
- ⅓ cup confectioner's sugar
- 14 oz Morello pitted cherries in syrup, drained and halved

For decoration

- 2.5 oz dark chocolate (60% – 70% cacao)
- 14-16 fresh ripe cherries

---

1. Pre-heat the oven to 350° F / 320° F fan.
2. Grease a 9inch spring form pan and line the base with baking paper.
3. Add the butter and sugar to a large mixing bowl and whisk together with an electric beater until fluffy and pale. Beat in the egg yolks one at a time, only adding the next when the current yolk has been incorporated.
4. In another bowl sift together the flour, baking powder, salt and cocoa powder. Fold the flour mixture into the butter mixture. Fold in the milk.
5. In a clean, dry bowl whisk the egg whites until soft peaks form. Gradually fold the egg whites into the batter until completely mixed.
6. Pour the batter into the prepared pan and gently smooth the surface of the batter using a spatula.
7. Bake in the pre-heated oven for 45 to 50 minutes, or until a wooden skewer or toothpick inserted into the middle of the sponge comes out clean. Remove from the oven and leave to cool for about 5 minutes before removing from the pan and placing on a wire rack to cool completely.

8. Cut the cake horizontally into 3 evenly-thick layers.
9. Whisk the cream together with the vanilla extract and confectioner's sugar until thick and voluminous, but still spreadable.
10. Place a sponge layer on the serving plate, sprinkle evenly with half the Kirschwasser and spread with half the jam. Evenly spread a thin layer of whipped cream over the jam using a palette knife. Evenly distribute half the Morello cherries onto the cream.
11. Place a layer of sponge on top and repeat with the remaining Kirschwasser and jam, another thin layer of cream and the remaining cherries.
12. Finely grate or scrape the chocolate into curls. Cover the top with chocolate and press chocolate around the side.
13. Pipe rosettes (small swirls) of whipped cream around the edge of the cake (they should just touch) and place a fresh cherry on each of them.

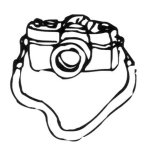

Torn Pancakes with Plum Compote

Kaiserschmarrn mit Zwetschgenkompott

Preparation time: **30 min**

Cooking time: **24 min**

Ingredients:

6 Servings

- 2 ½ cups all-purpose flour
- ¾ cup confectioner's sugar (about 3 ½ oz)
- ¼ tsp salt
- 1 cup milk
- 8 eggs, separated
- ½ tsp vanilla extract
- ½ cup raisins
- 2 tbsp light rum or orange liqueur
- 4 tbsp melted butter, or as needed
- ⅓ cup chopped nuts of choice
- confectioner's sugar for dusting

For the plum compote

- 1 lb. fresh plums (about 6 medium plums)
- 2 tbsp plum juice (or other berry juice), alternatively use water
- 1 cinnamon stick
- 2 – 3 tbsp sugar, or to taste (depends on sweetness of plums)
- ¼ tsp vanilla extract
- zest of 1 lemon
- 1 tbsp cornstarch or arrowroot (or as needed)
- 2 tbsp water

1. Pre-heat the oven to 140° F to warm serving plates and to keep the pancakes warm.
2. Soak the raisins in rum for about 30 minutes.
3. Sift the flour, sugar and salt into a large mixing bowl. Add the milk, egg yolks and vanilla. Beat with a hand mixer until smooth. Drain the raisins and stir into the batter.
4. In another clean bowl whisk the egg whites until soft peaks form. Using a spatula gently fold the egg whites into the batter until combined. Set aside to rest for 30 minutes.
5. Halve, pit and slice the plum halves into quarters. Add the plums, juice, cinnamon, sugar, vanilla and lemon zest to a saucepan. Bring to the boil and then reduce to a gentle simmer. Cover and simmer until the plums have broken down and are tender. Remove the cinnamon stick. Taste and add sugar if desired.

6. Dissolve the cornstarch in 2 tablespoons water. Slowly add to the plum compote, whisking constantly, until it has thickened to the desired consistency. You may not need all the cornstarch. Set aside.
7. Heat a tablespoon of butter in a non-stick pancake pan on medium heat. Pour in a ¼ of the batter, titling the pan to coat it evenly. Cook for 2 – 3 minutes, or until the underside is browned. Turn and finish cooking. Remove the pancake and tear into 1 ½ - 2-inch pieces using 2 spatulas. Place on a warm serving plate and keep warm in the oven.
8. Repeat and cook the remaining 3 pancakes.
9. Sprinkle the pancakes with chopped nuts, dust with confectioner's sugar and serve with plum compote. The compote can be served warm or at room temperature.

Cheesecake
Käsekuchen

Preparation time: **40 min + pastry chilling time**
Cooking time: **50 min**

Ingredients:

10 - 12 Servings

For the pastry

- 7 oz butter, chilled & diced
- ¾ cup confectioner's sugar
- ¼ tsp salt
- 1 large egg, beaten
- ½ tsp vanilla extract
- 2 ½ cups all-purpose flour
- flour for dusting counter surface

For the filling

- 1 cup granulated sugar
- ¾ cup all-purpose flour
- 7 tbsp milk
- 1 tsp vanilla extract
- 5 medium eggs, separated
- 4 cups quark (about 28 oz)
- zest of 1 lemon, grated
- 3 tbsp fresh lemon juice
- 1 cup whipping cream
- pinch of salt
- 3 tbsp cornstarch
- 1 cup confectioner's sugar

1. Preheat the oven to 340° F (fan).
2. Add all the pastry ingredients to a mixing bowl. Mix with a hand electric mixer, with the dough hook fitted, until you have a smooth dough. Squeeze into a ball and wrap with plastic wrap. Refrigerate for 2 hours.
3. Grease a 10-inch springform pan well with butter.
4. Dust a counter top with flour. Roll the pastry into a disc of 11 inches. Turn the pastry several times and dust the counter with flour, as necessary, to stop the pastry sticking to the counter top. Roll the pastry onto the rolling pin and lay over the springform pan. Lift and press the pastry down evenly over the base and push the sides up about an inch, pressing the pastry into the edge of the pan. Seal any holes that may appear.
5. Pierce the base all over with a fork. Line the base with a disc of parchment (kitchen) paper and cover with baking beans, dry beans

or rice. Blind bake for 15 – 18 minutes on a bottom shelf. Remove and set aside.

6. To a large mixing bowl add 1 cup granulated sugar, flour, milk and vanilla. Use an electric hand beater to whisk until well mixed. Whisk in the egg yolk, quark, lemon zest and lemon juice one after another and whisk until smooth. Stir in the cream.

7. Add the egg whites to a clean mixing bowl and add a pinch of salt. Whisk with an electric hand beater until stiff peaks form. Add the cornstarch and icing sugar and whisk for another 2 minutes.

8. Gently fold a third of the beaten egg whites into the quark mixture using a spatula. When blended, fold in the remaining beaten egg white.

9. Reduce the oven to 320° F.

10. Pour the quark mixture into the pre-baked pastry case. Smooth the top with a spatula.

11. Bake on a low shelf for 20 minutes. Remove from the oven and run a small, thin, sharp knife around the inside edge of the baking pan, about 1 inch deep down the side of the cake, being careful not to cut into the cake. To stop the knife from sticking to the cake moisten by dipping into a bowl of hot water. As you feel the knife sticking, again dip into hot water and rub off any batter that has stuck to the knife.

12. Return to the oven and bake for another 30 minutes. Turn the heat off and open the oven door slightly, about 2 inches or so. Leave to cool in the oven. You can check that the cake is cooked by inserting a wooden skewer into the center of the cake. If it comes out clean, it's done. If not bake for another 5 minutes and check again.

13. Once the oven is cool remove the cake to a wire rack to cool completely before removing from the springform pan.

14. Dust with confectioner's sugar before serving if desired.

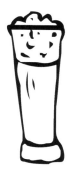

Hazelnut Waffles with hot Cherries & Raspberry Cream

Haselnusswaffeln mit heißen Kirschen & Himbeercreme

Preparation time: **20 min**
Cooking time: **22 min**

Ingredients:

6 Servings

For the waffles

- 9 tbsp (4.5 oz) butter, melted
- ½ cup granulated sugar
- ½ tsp vanilla extract
- 4 eggs
- ½ tsp lemon or orange zest, finely grated
- ⅔ cup all-purpose flour
- ½ cup cornstarch
- 2 tsp baking powder
- ½ tsp salt, or to taste
- ½ cup heavy cream
- ⅔ cup finely ground hazelnuts (about 3 ½ oz)

For the raspberry cream

- 2 ½ oz raspberries, fresh or frozen (about ½ cup)
- 1 ¼ cups full fat cream cheese or quark (about 11 oz)
- 5 tbsp raspberry jam, or to taste
- 2 tbsp confectioner's sugar
- 5 oz (1 cup) fresh raspberries (frozen raspberries are not suitable)

For the hot cherries

- 4 tbsp butter
- 6 tbsp superfine sugar, or to taste
- 1 tsp ground cinnamon
- 1 jar (24 oz) pitted sour cherries in light syrup
- syrup from drained cherries
- 1 tbsp fresh lemon juice, or to taste
- 1 – 2 tbsp arrowroot or cornstarch, as needed

1. Puree ½ cup of raspberries in a blender. Pass through a sieve to remove the seeds.
2. Add the raspberry puree, cream cheese, jam and confectioner's sugar to a bowl and mix until well combined. Set aside or refrigerate for later use.
3. Drain the cherries and reserve the liquid.
4. Melt the butter in a saucepan on medium heat. Stir in the sugar and cook until the sugar has melted and is lightly caramelized (browned).

Deglaze the saucepan with the reserved liquid from the cherries and stir in the cinnamon.

5. Stir in the cherries and taste. Add lemon juice to taste.
6. Dissolve the arrowroot/cornstarch in a little water. Slowly add to the saucepan, stirring constantly, until the sauce has thickened to a desired consistency. Simmer for another minute. If you have overthickened the sauce, loosen by adding a little water. Keep warm until the waffles are ready.
7. Add the butter and sugar to a mixing bowl and beat together using an electric hand beater. Add the vanilla, eggs and zest and beat until fluffy and well combined.
8. Sift together the flour, cornstarch, baking powder and salt. Gradually beat the flour mixture into the butter/sugar/egg mixture. Add the cream and beat in.
9. Fold in the ground hazelnuts until well mixed.
10. Prepare the waffles in the waffle-maker.
11. Dust the waffles with confectioner's sugar.
12. Serve with fresh raspberries, raspberry cream and hot cherries.

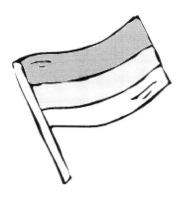

Apple Cake

Apfelkuchen

Preparation time: **20 min**

Cooking time: **45 min**

Ingredients:

6 – 8 Servings

- 2 large Bramley apples, cored & peeled
- 2 tbsp fresh lemon juice
- 2 cups all-purpose flour
- 2 tsp baking powder
- ½ tsp salt
- 5 oz butter, softened (½ cup + 2 tbsp)
- ¾ cup superfine sugar
- 3 eggs
- zest of 1 lemon, finely grated
- 5 tbsp whole milk
- 2 tbsp Demerara or light brown sugar
- ½ tsp cinnamon powder
- ½ cup sliced almonds
- confectioner's sugar for dusting (optional)

1. Pre-heat the oven to 300° F (fan).
2. Grease a 9-inch round cake pan with butter.
3. Cut the apples in half (through the cored hole) and slice into thin wedges. Toss in lemon juice to prevent them from oxidation.
4. Sift together the flour, baking powder and salt.
5. In another large bowl, whisk the butter and sugar together, using a hand electric beater, until fluffy and pale. Whisk in the eggs, one at a time. Add the flour mixture and lemon zest and mix well. Slowly add the milk, whisking well after each addition, until all the milk is incorporated and you have a smooth batter.
6. Pour the batter into the prepared cake pan and tap gently a few times on a counter top to settle the batter into the edges. Smooth the top with a spatula if necessary.
7. Arrange the apple wedges in a spiral / circle on top of the batter.
8. Toss together the Demerara sugar, cinnamon and almonds. Sprinkle evenly over the apple wedges.
9. Bake for 40 to 45 minutes, or until done and the top is golden brown. Test for doneness by inserting a skewer into the center of the cake. If it comes out clean, the cake is done. If not bake for another 5 minutes and test again.
10. Leave to cool in the pan for about 15 minutes.

11. Remove from the pan and cool on a wire rack. If necessary run a small, sharp knife around the inside edge of the pan to loosen the cake.
12. Serve warm or else cool completely and then dust with confectioner's sugar (optional).

Printed in Great Britain
by Amazon